# Delivering Your Placenta

## The Third Stage

Nadine Pilley Edwards

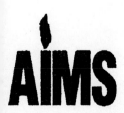

ASSOCIATION FOR IMPROVEMENTS IN THE MATERNITY SERVICES

# Acknowledgements

I would like to thank Sally Inch for all her work over many years on the third stage of labour and particularly for making this available and accessible to women.

I would also like to acknowledge the people who gave extremely generously of their time and knowledge to comment on the text. Beverley Beech, Alice Charlwood, Gill Gyte, Mandy Hawke, Louise Hulton, Elizabeth Key, Mavis Kirkham, Rosemary Mander, Jean Robinson, Christine Rodgers, Jane Rogers, Helen Shallow.

Gill Gyte in particular spent many hours discussing the finer details of the third stage of labour with me.

Nadine Pilley Edwards

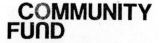

**COMMUNITY FUND**
lottery money making a difference

©AIMS September 1999

Published by AIMS on behalf of the British Maternity Trust

ISBN 1 874413 11 8

# Foreword

Work at AIMS means listening - listening in a way "which means you are prepared to be changed by what you hear". We never tire of hearing parents' stories of birth; each brings a new dimension. We are also enriched by listening to midwives and doctors telling us about their hands-on experience. As we read the latest *Confidential Enquiry* or randomised study, we hear the background music of these voices.

For the third stage of labour, the 'raw' consumer material is less plentiful than the feedback we get from parents on management of the first and second stages. Giving birth, and seeing and holding the new baby, are so overwhelming that for most mothers delivery of the placenta fades into the background unless something goes wrong. Cutting the cord may be most vividly spoken of by fathers, who are now often involved, and we had a deeply felt complaint from a father who was prevented from doing so. Most criticisms we receive about care shortly after delivery concentrate on handling of the baby and particularly on any separation from the mother, or exclusion of the father.

However, there are individual families, and especially those from certain cultures, for whom handling and disposal of the placenta is important, and lack of understanding or respect of their choices can be damaging.

Anyone who wants to learn about the consequences of cultural mismatch in medical care should read Anne Fadiman's brilliant and devastating account of a Hmong family in the USA - which includes their belief that the placenta should be buried under their hut - impossible to do in a city high rise apartment (Fadiman, 1997).

However, expectant parents often tell us that one of their concerns is the cord not being cut too soon - though we have no idea how common knowledge or anxiety about this is. Whether of not the baby is getting all the blood it should have for the best start in life is a simple enough question for parents to understand. This is a prime example of an issue parents will not question if they do not know about it, since they assume professionals know best. But once they have information, they immediately grasp its importance, whatever their level of education.

We continue to receive a steady trickle of complaints about retained parts of placenta not being detected before mothers are sent home, and the subsequent problems they have. Sometimes diagnosis or treatment of infection are delayed, and women may have prolonged ill health. This is nothing to do with active or physiological management, but basic quality of care in inspecting the placenta after delivery to ensure that it is complete.

There are also women who were traumatised or upset by manual removal of the placenta. One vividly described floating above her body and could describe what was done and said in theatre, and could describe a doctor she had never met, even though she was under general anaesthetic at the time. She suffered severe post-traumatic stress disorder.

Unlike the widespread outcry on induction and augmentation of labour, and fetal heart monitoring, consumer challenge to routine third stage management has come almost entirely from those who have more background and knowledge - the organised maternity groups like AIMS and the NCT, but we were not alone. We were allied with many midwives, and some doctors, who were asking similar questions. Would there have been a randomised trial of physiological versus active management of the third stage without consumer pressure? Throughout the discussions there has been a continual to-ing and fro-ing and sharing ideas between ourselves and professionals.

It simply became a natural extension of the questions we had learned to ask from the 70s when induction rates soared. Why interfere with Nature routinely when you can do more harm that good? What outcomes are you measuring? For whose good are you intervening - the good of the mother, the baby, the staff or the institution? Do these research studies actually prove the benefits they claim, and who defines them as benefits? Were adverse effects effectively sought and measured?

The primary justification for third stage intervention, of course, is prevention of post-partum haemorrhage. Fortunately there were only five maternal deaths from PPH in three years covering the latest *Confidential Enquiry into Maternal Deaths* 1994-6 (Department of Health, 1998). Four of them followed caesarean section and the remaining one happened after vacuum extraction. There were no deaths following normal delivery. However for other causes of haemorrhage - placenta praevia ( three deaths, two of them associated with embedded placentas with a previous uterine scar) and placental abruption (four deaths) - risks are increased if the mother has a previous caesarean section.

So is the risk of haemorrhage from placenta accreta (embedded placenta) increased when manual removal is attempted, or at a later caesarean? (Zaki, 1998; Hemminki, 1996). The current high rate of caesareans is creating a population of mothers at future risk of antenatal and postnatal haemorrhage, as well as rupture of the uterus. Unfortunately when deaths associated with a previous uterine scar occur, the Confidential Enquiry do not investigate how necessary the earlier caesarean was when they are judging the avoidability of death.

However what AIMS hears about most is delayed diagnosis of heavy blood loss, and late or inadequate treatment, and prolonged low physical and emotional health afterwards. It is interesting that almost all of these cases involve haemorrhage from trauma - from unsuspected injury, from episiotomy or tears. Is it possible that the midwife's confidence in routine Syntometrine reduces awareness and watchfulness? Even more worrying are the occasional stories we get about an almost deliberate refusal to diagnose or record heavy blood loss which seem similar to staff refusals to admit that women have had serious postnatal sepsis. *"If we don't see it and record it, it didn't happen"* seems to be the philosophy.

Quantity of blood loss, the accuracy of estimations, and what constitutes a "haemorrhage" rather than "normal" loss - these are still unsettled questions. One doctor routinely estimated "499 mls" - presumably to keep within the common British definition that more than 500 mls constituted a haemorrhage (Logue, 1990). If he had been in Holland, where the definition is apparently 1000 ml, he could have gone up to 999 mls! As we explain these problems to parents, many of them are astonished at how inaccurate and unscientific expert maternity care can be. But they talk about the soaked mattress, the pools of blood on the floor, and no-one listening to them and how long mothers took to recover from the birth. The danger here comes not from lack of active management, which they received, but from staff who were not caring and paying attention.

No-one mentions how the behaviour of individual accouchers can affect risk. Margaret Logue's important, but little known, study showed that some obstetricians caused twelve times the haemorrhage rate of others - related to their personality - and that midwives too have varying rates (Logue, 1990). Does this mean that Syntometrine needs to be used when some staff are on duty but not others? If her study at one hospital showed such a marked effect, we wonder what analysis of outcomes at other hospitals would show.

What is clear from mothers' comments is that doctors and midwives who cause physical blood loss are also likely to cause emotional damage, and women are just as vulnerable to psychic trauma during the third stage as at other stages of labour.

When randomised trials report on outcome from any extra intervention, they do not mention the additional risks each one brings. With every drug comes a risk that it will be given to the wrong person in the wrong dose or at the wrong time. And drugs given by injection are riskier than those given orally, since their diverse effects are likely to be more severe, and they can be injected into the wrong place as well as the wrong person. For additional procedures, each new intake of staff has to practise and learn on someone - like the mother whose cord was broken when the medical student was told to practise controlled cord traction.

Those of us who often dip into medical literature, soon realise that adverse effects of intervention often surface only when a different treatment becomes available for comparison. Proponents or producers of the new drug or treatment will then happily write about the disadvantages of the old, in order to convert colleagues to the new. This is also true of different oxytocic drugs used to reduce haemorrhage risk in the third stage.

There are still many unanswered questions. One midwife told us that Syntometrine may reduce immediate blood loss, but that loss may simply come later, when it does not count as PPH. Another suggests that pharmaceutical use of oxytocin may reduce mothers' own ability to produce natural oxytocin in subsequent deliveries. These are interesting, but unresearched issues.

In debates on the third stage once again we are involved in argument about time in labour. Who defines "normal" time for natural processes and who controls it? This is illustrated in a social study of midwifery: *"Even Syntometrine was said to be used in the third stage of labour 'to shorten the third stage' as if there was some urgency to end this undesirable condition."* (Hunt and Symonds, 1995). Later the authors refer to the speed with which women are "washed and warded" after delivery: *"The staff have been very efficient but perhaps they were not effective. The urgency to complete the process had overtaken everything else."*

In this booklet, Nadine Edwards, AIMS' Vice Chair, summarises what we know and do not know about research on the third stage and highlights some of the issues of concern to parents and professionals alike.

**Jean Robinson**
Research Officer, AIMS

# Introduction

The third stage of labour marks the final stage of the awesome transition from woman to mother. For most women or parents this is a particularly precious moment, as they meet their baby for the first time face to face.

*'Yet, for the mother, this is the most dangerous stage of labour'* (Sleep 1993)

This could be said to sum up the medical approach to the third stage of labour, and whilst there may be some truth in it, approaches to health based largely on fear are not always logical or designed to work in the best interests of mother and child.

It is, of course, in the privileged context of a developed, relatively affluent society that this booklet is written. On a global scale, we have the enormous advantage, that few women and babies die in childbirth - though of the few women who do, excessive blood loss (postpartum haemorrhage or PPH) after birth is still implicated (Lewis 1998). We do however have the disadvantage that birth in most parts of the western world has become increasingly medicalised, and some women and babies suffer the side-effects of the overuse of medication and medical procedures, with both its known and unknown effects.

This booklet is for parents and midwives who would like to know more about the third stage of labour, why there are ongoing discussions about the benefits and drawbacks of managing the third stage of labour or letting nature take its course, and what research and experience can tell us about the birth of the placenta.

The third stage of labour is usually defined as the period immediately following the baby's birth until the placenta and membranes have been born (Sweet 1997). Also described as the time 'when the activity and excitement accompanying the birth of the baby are replaced by the parents' quiet and wonderous contemplation of their offspring. The focus shifts from the mother's concentrated exertions to the miracle of the newborn. There is a sense of emotional and physical relief.' (Sleep 1993).

The main discussion focuses on the active and physiological approaches to the third stage of labour. In essence, active management of the third stage involves a care-giver intervening in some way to bring about the birth of the placenta and a physiological approach allows nature to take its course. Whilst there are different definitions of these, broadly speaking, active management includes: the midwife giving the woman an intramuscular injection of an oxytocic drug as the baby is being born or immediately after birth; clamping and cutting the cord immediately after birth; and applying gentle traction to the woman's end of the cord to birth the placenta reasonably quickly. The physiological approach usually means that the third stage occurs naturally, without the use of ocytocic drugs. The cord is left unclamped and uncut, until it has stopped pulsating or until the placenta is born. The placenta is then birthed by the woman's own efforts and may take longer than when active management is used.

This booklet includes a brief history of the third stage of labour, explains the differences between active and physiological approaches to the third stage, discusses the research on this issue, examines other views about the third stage of labour and looks at how women may decide to have a managed or physiological third stage, given the complexities of this topic.

# Historical Background

It has been suggested that in early biblical writings on childbirth, no mention is made of third stage problems such as postpartum haemorrhage and retained placenta (where the placenta does not come out). Whilst this does not necessarily mean that there were no problems, midwife and author, Sally Inch (1989) suggests that problems may have been exacerbated by some of the interventions to the third stage of labour, introduced in more recent history. This is reflected in other writings (Priya 1992, Dunn 1991, Botha 1968).

It seems that, as the third stage of labour became increasingly managed, cord cutting was one of the first interventions to become normal practice. It has been suggested that this was so that the baby could be removed from the bed and the attendants could focus on the mother unhindered (Inch 1989). It is thought that because the quantity of blood escaping from the placental end of the cut cord could make a considerable mess, the practice of clamping the cord was developed (Inch 1989). In a comprehensive review of third stage management, in her publication *Birthrights* Sally Inch (1989) quotes Montgomery's view that these interventions might be due to the fact that:

*"As the physician became more skilful with the use of haemostats, scissors and ligatures, the umbilical cord presented an inviting site for surgical procedures, and the present custom of immediate severance and immediate ligation, of the cord followed. Ligation of the cord makes it possible to get babies and mothers out of the delivery room more rapidly, just as low forceps contribute to more rapid care. Whether they have added to the ultimate welfare of the newborn is a question"* (Inch 1989).

Montgomery's question continues to be pertinent and could still be applied to many aspects of maternity care. With notable exceptions, it is a question which appears to have been largely overlooked in modern obstetrics.

The third stage of labour continued to be more systematically managed as medical men involved themselves more regularly in childbirth from the 18th and 19th centuries onwards. At this time and until relatively recently, many women suffered from poverty and ill-health, gave birth many times and could not afford enough nourishing food. Postpartum haemorrhage was therefore more common and its effects devastating. It was second only to infection as a cause of maternal death. The introduction of Ergometrine in 1935 was seen as a welcome breakthrough and was originally given intravenously to stop active bleeding.

Ergot is a fungus found on rotting rye and its ability to produce contractions of the uterus following birth has been known for centuries. It was used by midwives in the 17th and 18th centuries, but was used cautiously because of its inclination to cause gangrene. It was first introduced into obstetric practice in 1807 but did not become popular until its reintroduction in 1932. By 1935 a new water-soluble ergot principle had been isolated which became known as Ergometrine).

Given intravenously after birth, Ergometrine works within 45 seconds and is extremely effective, but is not without its side-effects - most notably of causing retained placentas (Begley 1990). Nevertheless, like many other obstetric procedures, it began to be used more frequently as a 'just in case' measure to prevent excessive bleeding. (For more detailed information about its history see van Dongen & de Groot 1995 and Inch 1989).

In 1954, it was thought that some of the side-effects of Ergometrine, especially that of causing retained placentas may have been solved by the manufacture of a synthetic, oxytocic drug (one which causes contractions of the uterus), Syntocinon.

However, Syntocinon was not considered to be as effective as Ergometrine, and subsequently, Syntometrine was developed in the 1960s. This combines Ergometrine and Syntocinon and is commonly used today. From then on, it has generally been assumed to be necessary and desirable for all birthing women to be given one of these drugs to expel the placenta after birth.

Discussion since then has tended to focus on which drug is preferred for third stage management, and the optimum time to give it, rather than question the necessity for drugs to be routinely given. A number of studies have looked into how the placenta might be delivered most efficiently, comparing the outcome of related procedures such as controlled cord traction (pulling on the cord), maternal effort (the woman pushing the placenta out herself) and fundal pressure (pressing on the womb). Less attention has been paid to what measures, if any, might reduce the likelihood of postpartum haemorrhage occurring in the first place.

# Natural Birth of the Placenta

The uterine muscle is unique in its elasticity during pregnancy and its ability to retract and contract during labour and birth. The volume of blood flowing through the placenta in any one minute is 500-800 mls (Sleep 1993). As the uterus contracts and retracts during the third stage of labour, causing the placenta to separate from the uterine wall, this flow of blood ceases almost simultaneously.

After the birth, if the third stage is not interfered with, fetal blood flows from the placenta through the cord to the baby. This is thought to be linked to expansion of lung circulation in the baby (Gyte, personal communication). Strong uterine contractions cause the uterine wall to contract making the placenta peel away. As this blood moves from the placenta, the placenta becomes more compact. It peels away from the uterine wall, usually from the centre or sometimes slides off from an edge (Sleep 1993).

The placenta, when it peels from the centre, folds in on itself and the contracting upper part of the uterus causes it to fall into the lower segment. Simultaneously the muscle fibres in the upper segment (sometimes referred to as 'living ligatures') are able to clamp the torn uterine blood vessels due to the pressure of the rapidly shrinking uterus.

**16**

# THE PLACENTA

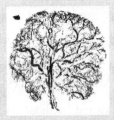

Women may be interested to know that the placenta is roughly the size of a dinner plate, that it usually weighs about a sixth to a fifth of the baby's weight, that the length of the umbilical cord is 50cms on average. Many women are unaware that the placenta is their property. A woman should be consulted antenatally, about its disposal. Occasionally women are distressed to learn subsequently that they could have kept it and disposed of it as they wished.

In the past, placentas were used in cosmetics, but are now usually disposed of by incineration. In some areas, blood is drained from the placenta and cord and used in research or in the treatment of some diseases. There is a growing interest in this extraordinary organ, which nourishes the baby during pregnancy.

There is also growing interest in the rituals surrounding the placenta in other cultures (Priya 1992). Some parents are redeveloping their own rituals in Britain - for example, planting a tree, bush or plant over the placenta. Occasionally, a woman may cook and eat her placenta (as shown on a recent cookery programme on television) in an attempt to avoid postnatal depression due to the hormones contained in it, or just because of its nourishing qualities.

Meanwhile the cervix remains open and, as the placenta meets no resistance it falls into the vagina and is expelled, sometimes aided, as Kierse (1998) suggests, by the woman's pushing efforts, gravity or nipple stimulation.

French obstetrician, Michel Odent (1998b) believes that when labour and birth have been normal, without induction or acceleration of labour with synthetic hormones, without pharmaceutical pain relief, without instrumental delivery, and the woman can remain undisturbed and adopt whatever position she pleases, there is usually no need to induce or accelerate birth of the placenta either. While there is no bleeding there is no need for haste. Whether or not complications arise depends on a variety of factors.

The woman's general health and whether or not she is anaemic are important. The progress of the first and second stages of labour and whether she has developed ketosis (ketones in blood or urine), or hypotonic (ineffective) uterine action, or become exhausted can all have an impact on the third stage. The skill of those attending the birth in detecting developing problems, preventing or treating a postpartum haemorrhage, protecting the woman from infection, detecting retained placenta and preventing or treating shock are equally important. One of the main risks seems to be the lack of knowledge as to what constitutes safe practice for a physiological third stage of labour.

For example, in one study (Featherstone 1999) using one particular definition of a physiological third stage, only 33% of a group of midwives appeared to understand physiological third stage. According to Featherstone, when describing their practice, 10% described, unknowingly, potentially unsafe practices (such as omitting giving an oxytocic drug, but then applying all other components of active management) during a physiological third stage, which may increase the likelihood of excessive bleeding during physiological third stage.

Based on his own work and observation, Odent suggests that certain principles may positively facilitate the birth of the placenta, and at the same time enhance crucial bonding processes between mother and baby. These occur because of the release of certain hormones - most notably, oxytocin, commonly known as the "love hormone". They can only occur however, if the mother and baby are in a warm room, and there is undisturbed contact between them. He believes that quietness and privacy are essential (Odent 1998a, Odent 1998b).

Typically the third stage is said to last around 5-15 minutes when it is actively managed (Sleep 1993). This can be longer when the process is not artificially speeded up and up to one and a half hours is considered within the normal range by some (Cronk & Flint 1989). There has been debate over the years about the optimum length of time for the third stage. Whilst some have recommended waiting one hour to reduce the number of retained

**19**

placentas, others have suggested that the third stage should be left only half an hour as the rate of postpartum haemorrhage rises after that time.

There are descriptions involving wide variations. One account describes a breech baby arriving unexpectedly at home, wearing its placenta like a 'floppy hat' (Wesson 1990), whilst other anecdotal accounts tells of the placenta being born many hours after the baby's birth - in one case, 48 hours. One midwife researcher suggests that she knows of no sound evidence to intervene after an hour if time is not a constraint and that the decision to intervene after one hour is often a purely pragmatic decision in busy maternity units. (Rogers 1999, personal communication).

# Actively Managed Third Stage

Active management of the third stage of labour is routinely recommended in nearly all hospitals in the UK. It is considered by most medical and many midwifery professionals to reduce blood loss and shorten the third stage. In the author's experience, women often report that midwives attending births in the community, tend to have a more flexible approach to this issue. Over the last decade, a growing number of researchers, midwives and parents have questioned whether or not active management of the third stage of labour should be routine for *all* women. Some have suggested that the woman's individual health and circumstances should be taken into account and that the effects of oxytocic drugs and other components of active management on the woman and baby should be given more consideration.

Syntometrine is a powerful oxytocic substance which stimulates uterine contractions. It is still, usually the drug of choice for third stage management in the UK (though syntocinon is increasingly being used as an alternative). It is typically administered by injection, intramuscularly, into the upper, outer part of the woman's buttock as the baby's anterior shoulder is born - though there are variations on this. This is to make sure that it begins to take effect as soon as the baby is born. A 1ml vial of Syntometrine is made up of 5 units of syntocinon and 0.5mg. of Ergometrine. The former acts when given intramuscularly within 2.5 minutes, and the latter within 6-7 minutes.

This combined preparation results in strong rhythmic contractions, followed minutes later by a stronger, more sustained contraction which lasts several hours. Thus, in order to avoid a retained placenta it has been assumed that it needs to be delivered within a relatively short length of time. Otherwise it must be removed manually, in which case the woman will need a spinal or a general anaesthetic. These can entail disadvantages to the woman's health and her ability to bond with, feed and generally care for her baby immediately after birth - in practice manual removals are not usually carried out for an hour or so after birth.

It has been suggested that the cervix will sometimes eventually relax and open of its own accord to allow birth of the placenta if the above occurs (Cronk & Flint 1989) - though this is not common practice in Britain.

When the third stage is actively managed, the cord is usually clamped and cut immediately after the baby's birth and the midwife then places her hand lightly on the mother's abdomen to await a contraction. She may place a container under the woman to catch and assess blood loss and use a specific manoeuvre - controlled cord traction (CCT) to ensure rapid delivery of the placenta once there are signs of placental separation. This involves sustained traction on the cord, whilst applying counter-pressure to the uterus. The woman is usually lying down, or in a semi-reclining position as it is then easier for her attendants to apply the different components of active management.

One study suggested that before applying CCT, it is advantageous to wait until the cord has lengthened and a fresh trickle of blood has been noticed, which indicates that the placenta has separated from the uterine wall (Levy & Moore 1985).

# Oxytocic Drugs

Undoubtedly, oxytocic drugs have saved many lives and will continue to do so. They are effective in dealing with postpartum haemorrhage in most cases. As mentioned, Ergometrine works within 45 seconds if given intravenously and almost always stops active bleeding, though is not usually used on its own, or given intravenously in Britain, because of associated problems. Syntometrine works as detailed above, and is also almost always successful in stopping blood loss. It is not, however, appropriate for women with pre-existing high blood pressure, in which case one of its two components, Syntocinon, can be used on its own.

There is now growing evidence to suggest that there are advantages to using Syntocinon on its own rather than Syntometrine. In research carried out by McDonald et al (1993) it remained unclear what dose should be used, though 10iu could be more effective than 5iu. It seems that intramuscular Syntocinon is slightly less protective against moderate blood loss, but has none of the potentially serious side effects of Syntometrine (McDonald et al 1999; see also Anderson 1998 and Anderson 1999 for further comment).

In cases of persistent bleeding, where Syntometrine has failed to stop bleeding, prostaglandins (similar to those used in second stage

**23**

management - see AIMS booklet *Birthing Your Baby - The Second Stage* for more information on risks and benefits) are effective (Peyser & Kupfenninc 1990). In these circumstances their use is still recommended (Gulmezoglu 1998) though research is currently examining the use of a drug called Misoprostol. This could prove to be a safer, more stable and cheaper drug and can be given in tablet form.

A large international, multicentre, randomised controlled trial, co-ordinated by the World Health Organisation started in April 1998 (Gumezoglu 1998) in order to examine the use of Misoprostol. This trial was ongoing at time of writing.

In the earlier 1990s, in their conclusion about third stage management, the authors of the first edition of the *Guide to Effective Care in Pregnancy and Childbirth* stated that the routine use of Syntometrine reduces the risk of haemorrhage by as much as 30-40% (Enkin et al 1991). The most recent edition reached similar conclusions but was a little more cautious about the advantages of active management of the third stage (Enkin et al 1995). An updated, third edition should be published in late 1999. One of the conclusions of the most up to date systematic review of third stage trials supported these earlier conclusions, that blood loss is reduced when the third stage of labour is managed (Prendiville et al 1999).

Research is however rather mixed in its findings, but a number of studies show reduced blood loss associated with routine use of this drug (Rogers et al 1998, Prendiville et al 1988). See also a review by Dewhurst (1990). On the other hand, there are a number of studies showing other results and there are other views on the disadvantages and side effects associated with the use of Syntometrine for healthy women experiencing normal labours (Prichard et al 1995, Thilaganathan 1993, Begley 1990, Inch 1983, Ward, 1983 Botha, 1968). For example:

- it necessitates further interventions which have inherent risks of their own, such as early cutting of the cord and CCT. In addition, it involves the woman and her midwife in a race against the clock to birth the placenta before the cervix closes

- Syntometrine does not prevent all cases of haemorrhage as there are other reasons for bleeding during the third stage. Episiotomies have been known to be the cause of a postpartum haemorrhage (see Inch 1989 for further comment)

- Ergometrine may, on occasion, cause retained placentas (Begley 1990) - though recent research has not found this to be the case with Syntometrine (Rogers et al 1998)

- common side effects include nausea, vomiting, headaches, tingling of the limbs, dizziness, ringing in the ears, palpitations, pains in the back and legs and raised blood pressure (Inch 1989).

- very rare complications include cardiac arrest (heart failure), intracerebral haemorrhage (bleeding in the brain), myocardial infarction (heart attack), postpartum eclampsia (high blood pressure and possible fits after birth), pulmonary oedema (fluid on the lungs) and, in some rare cases, these have led to the woman's death (see Inch 1989)

- though extremely rare now, intrauterine asphyxia (lack of oxygen) may occur when an undiagnosed twin is present because the Syntometrine is given with the anterior shoulder of the first baby - the death rate for the second twin is 35%, and few escape unscathed (Inch 1989). The use of scans has reduced this unusual incidence, but it has occurred in a hospital in Britain recently as reported in the national press

- though very rare, injections can be mixed up. Neonatal convulsions were caused in a baby given an oxytocic drug instead of Vitamin K. At least one baby has died when a mother was given Syntometrine instead of pethidine during the first stage of labour

- if the cord is left unclamped and Syntometrine is given during the birth of the baby's anterior shoulder, the baby receives more than its physiological quota of blood as the uterus clamps down strongly, forcing blood very rapidly through the cord. The baby may appear over-transfused, pink and shiny, and experience slight breathing difficulties (Dunn 1973). Although there is no published research, over-transfusion is thought by some to be a reason for the rise in numbers of babies with 'physiological jaundice'. On the other hand if the cord is clamped immediately after birth, the baby does not receive its full quota of blood, and appears slightly limp and pale (Dunn 1973). It can take up to 6 weeks for the baby to regain a normal iron count (see Sleep 1993). As yet, the significance of this remains unknown

- in some countries it is considered bad practice to give oxytocic drugs before the birth of the placenta, as this is thought to cause problems, such as retained placentas. Oxytocic drugs are given after the birth of the placenta

- Syntometrine affects smooth muscle and where it is given as the baby is being born, whilst the cord is still intact, it reaches the baby. It is thought by some commentators that it might be implicated in causing the well-known 'three month colic'

- a recent study showed that women who did not receive Ergometrine during the third stage breastfed for longer periods (Begley 1990). This seemed to be specific to this study where Ergometrine was given intravenously for the third stage of labour. As previously mentioned, recent research suggests that Syntocinon may be a better option as it has fewer side effects and does not appear to affect breastfeeding rates

# Cord Cutting and Clamping

The cord is usually clamped in two places and then cut between the two clamps immediately after the baby's birth. This makes it easier for the midwife to apply controlled cord traction (see page 32 for discussion about this practice), to make sure the placenta is born reasonably quickly. Whenever the cord is cut, it should be cut 3-4 cms away from the baby's body to avoid pinching the skin or clamping a portion of the gut which may rarely protrude into the cord. A swab should be held over the cord to avoid spraying of blood.

It has been suggested that, in days gone by it would have been unnatural for a mother to cut the umbilical cord quickly. She would have been unlikely to have anything with which to cut it, and could not have easily moved herself and her baby before the birth of the placenta. (In the animal world the cord remains untouched after birth and is then severed some time later).

Obstetrician, MC Botha observed 26,000 births over a ten year period among the Bantu women in Africa (Botha 1968). These women give birth in a squatting position and the cord is left completely untouched until after the birth of the placenta and membranes. Although he said that he saw many complications during this time he seldom witnessed a retained placenta and a blood transfusion was never given for a postpartum haemorrhage. British professor in perinatal medicine, Peter Dunn, during his extensive work in the field of third stage management made similar observations (Dunn 1991). A Dutch doctor argued that nature cannot usually be improved upon and attempts to do so without cause can be detrimental to mother and child (Kloosterman 1975).

Early clamping and cutting of the umbilical cord may have a number of undesirable side-effects, including:

- reducing the volume of blood the baby receives by 75-125 mls., especially if the cord is clamped within the first minute of birth (see Prendiville and Elbourne 1989 and Inch, 1983). This is also suggested by the results of the Bristol (Prendiville et al 1988) and Hinchingbrooke (Rogers et al, 1998) trials. This may result in lower iron stores in the baby.

- research has shown the placenta to be bulkier when fetal blood was not allowed to pass to the baby (Dunn et al 1966) - this might prolong placental separation due to fetal blood remaining in the placenta which may delay retraction

- increasing blood loss (Botha 1968) - though there is little robust evidence on this issue, midwife Valerie Levy suggests that clamping the maternal end of the cord may interfere with placental separation and predispose a woman to a blood loss (Levy 1992)

- severing the baby's lifeline quickly and suddenly - especially crucial if the baby is premature (particularly if born by caesarean section) or slow to breathe (Dunn 1991, Dunn 1989). Some alternative therapists believe that, even for the healthy newborn, this is a shock

- increasing the possibility of feto-maternal transfusion (mixing of the baby and mother's blood) because of a larger volume of blood remaining in the placenta. Pressure is exerted as the uterus attempts to contract to expel the placenta. This pressure can cause placental vessels to rupture, allowing fetal cells into the maternal system. This may be critical if the mother is Rhesus negative and her baby is positive (Lapido, 1971). Rogers et al (1998) considered this in their research but did not confirm an association. However, removing the clamp from the maternal end of the cord (as done in their trial) has been shown to decrease feto-maternal transfusion

- it is suggested by Inch (1989) that when blood in the placenta is not given time to drain because of clamping the cord quickly and leaving it clamped at the maternal end, there is the possibility that extra blood clots will form in the woman, providing an ideal environment for infection. She and Sleep (1993) suggest that stagnant blood may also be left in the stump of the baby's cord which provides another place for infection to develop - though a subclinical (mild) degree of infection of the cord stump is normal and is thought to facilitate its separation. On the other hand, Rogers et al (1998) did not find this to be the case

- interference with delicate and complex changes in the baby's heart and circulatory systems which has been linked to idiopathic respiratory distress (breathing difficulties for no apparent reason) and may be crucial for a premature baby, or a baby whose breathing is already depressed (see Dunn 1989 and Inch, 1983 for detailed comment)

It is assumed that most healthy babies tolerate active management of the third stage. Though it has been suggested that there may be implications as mentioned above, as well as issues not yet thought about, both in the short and long-term, for women and babies (Odent 1998b). This needs further research.

There are a number of specific advantages associated with delaying clamping of the cord, as follows:

- the woman and her baby can remain undisturbed to allow the natural physiological processes which cause placental separation and enhance relationship forming between mother and infant to occur unhindered

- the placenta continues to function, carrying oxygen to the baby after birth. This may be advantageous, particularly if the baby is premature or asphyxiated (Dunn 1985). Anecdotal evidence from midwives suggests that less resuscitation may be required if cords were left alone after birth

- it has been suggested that the cord may separate more rapidly postnatally (see Sleep 1993)

- the baby receives its full quota of blood, which may be as much as 40% of the circulating volume and is important in maintaining haematocrit levels (ratio of red blood cells to total volume of blood) (Yao & Lind 1974)

# Controlled Cord Traction

Sometimes known as CCT, this action involves the midwife applying traction to the cord with one hand and guarding the woman's uterus with her other hand and is one of the components of active management of the third stage of labour. It is believed to contribute to a shorter third stage and is applied as the Syntocinon (on its own, or with Ergometrine) causes a strong uterine contraction following the baby's birth.

Problems associated with the use of CCT include:

- the risk of pulling out an incompletely separated placenta

- the cord very occasionally being snapped or pulled off. This could be critical if Syntometrine or Ergometrine had been given and there were any delay in the third stage

- the risk of causing the uterus to invert partially or fully. This is a very rare event which can also happen when oxytocics have not been used for the third stage, but is more common when CCT is used (Inch 1989)

- causing the woman pain if the placenta is not completely separarted

However the third stage is managed, any pressing, pushing or other handling of the uterus ('fundus fiddling') can be dangerous and painful and occasionally cause bleeding. It should be avoided and not confused with gentle massage of the uterus when it does not contract, or relaxes again following birth

# A Physiological Third Stage

This is sometimes also referred to as 'passive' or 'expectant' management of the third stage of labour. There appear to be important advantages to this approach for healthy women experiencing normal labour, including:

- avoiding all the disadvantages (real and potential) to women and babies associated with active management of the third stage (see above)

- eliminating the sense of urgency and anxiety about birthing the placenta within the time frame associated with active management

- a calm and quiet atmosphere can be maintained, once the baby is born, rather than one of action. This enables everyone present to appreciate and experience the wonder of birth and to welcome the new baby. Undisturbed, the mother who is focusing on the baby in her arms, is able to enjoy skin-to-skin and eye contact. She will thus be in the best possible hormonal balance to stimulate the necessary release of natural oxytocin (a hormone that makes the uterus contract) to expel the placenta (Odent 1998b)

- the woman's sense of confidence in her own body may be enhanced

If a physiological third stage is to be considered as an option by women and midwives it is important that:

- the woman and midwife should fully understand the normal physiology of the first, second and third stages of labour and understand the benefits and disadvantages of both managed and expectant approaches to the third stage

- third stage is discussed antenatally, and that a flexible approach is adopted by the woman and her midwife

- the woman is enabled to adopt the positions she finds most comfortable. Odent (1998b) suggests that women will usually lie down after birth and should not be instructed to be upright - though this is contrary to advice often given to women, which suggests that upright positions harness the use of gravity

- labour or birth has not been induced or augmented using oxytocic drugs, or interfered with in any other way

- the woman and midwife recognise the benefits of putting the baby to the breast (but that this is not a prerequisite for a natural third stage).

- the midwife recognises the signs of placental separation and descent, and is sensitive to the possible causes when placental separation seems to be delayed. (If the baby is not yet ready to feed, some midwives suggest that nipple stimulation may help promote the release of oxytocin.) Just as in earlier phases of labour, emotional factors might be delaying the process and the woman may need patience and quietness to let the placenta go, and make the final transition to motherhood. It is important that she does not feel observed by those around her (Odent 1998b)

The woman should be kept warm and comfortable, as blood loss is associated with higher levels of catecholamines (stress hormones). The woman produces these if she is too cool (see Odent 1998b for further comment).

It may also be reassuring for the woman to know beforehand, that when she breastfeeds her baby, the natural oxytocin released causes her uterus to contract.

For more detailed information about the physiology of the separation and expulsion of the placenta, and the different components of active and passive approaches to the third stage of labour, a number of midwives with a particular interest in this aspect of labour and birth have written informative chapters in midwifery textbooks and books for women. See for example Sweet (1997), Sleep (1993), Levy (1990) and Inch (1989).

# Expectant vs. Active Management - The Bristol Third Stage Trial

Until 1986 results of research into third stage management remained contradictory and confusing. With this in mind, researchers planned and executed a large trial at Bristol Maternity Hospital. This was designed to show whether or not active management of the third stage should be routinely recommended to all women (Prendiville et al 1988).

The results of the trial were published in the British Medical Journal in 1988 and were considered to be authoritative and definitive by many doctors and midwives. The authors concluded that active management should continue to be routinely recommended, as blood loss in the women receiving physiological management was significantly higher.

Criticisms of the Bristol trial appeared in both professional and lay journals following the publication of the results. It was pointed out that Bristol Maternity Hospital had a policy of recommending routine active management of the third stage and that, prior to the trial, only six weeks had been allocated for the midwives to become familiar and confident in using a physiological approach.

One of the criticisms appeared to be that women at increased risk of bleeding were included in the trial and that active management for all women was recommended, without considering whether or not physiological third stage might be appropriate for healthy women following physiological labours and births.

Other criticisms of the Bristol study included that:

- the midwives may have lacked experience and confidence in physiological third stage management due to the short time allowed for training. There is ongoing debate about whether or not this affects outcomes (Featherstone 1999, Kierse 1998, Stockdale 1997)

- women in the physiological arm of the trial had, in some cases, not experienced normal first and second stages of labour, which may have made them more likely to suffer excessive blood loss after birth

- women at known risk of postpartum haemorrhage were not excluded from the trial, although women with high blood pressure were selected out of the group receiving Syntometrine

- a large number of women (53%) who should have had physiological third stages had neither physiological or active management. They received a mixed approach including components of active management such as clamping the cord and early cord cutting. In some cases, a physiological approach seemed only to mean inappropriately avoiding the use of Syntometrine (Gyte 1991, Gyte 1990, Inch 1990, Stevenson, 1989). Other measures used on their own can increase the risk of excessive bleeding

It is interesting to note that both women and midwives involved in the trial preferred active management of the third stage (Harding et al 1989), though perhaps this is not surprising considering the high rate of problems in the physiological group. Also, because the Bristol Trial was a randomised controlled trial (RCT), women who had already stated a preference about the third stage of labour were automatically excluded from the trial. More recent research suggested that women were satisfied with whichever form of third stage management they received (Rogers et al 1998).

This appears to support the notion that 'what is must be best' (Porter & MacIntyre 1984) and that many women assume that any care offered must have been well thought out (Santalaahti et al 1998) In this trial too, women who intended to have a natural third stage were excluded from the trial. It would be interesting to know if the woman's expressed choice has any bearing on outcomes.

Critics of the Bristol trial were criticised in turn. The evidence to show that induction or acceleration with oxytocic drugs in labour predispose women to postpartum haemorrhage, and that the position of the woman or early cord clamping might affect outcome were questioned (Chalmers 1990).

Posture during the third stage of labour was not found to affect blood loss in the more recent Hinchingbrooke trial (Rogers et al 1998) and Odent (1998b) suggests that women would usually choose to lie down after giving birth.

When the trial was carried out, physiological third stage was a relatively new concept. The Bristol trial was important in raising questions, which subsequent research has attempted to follow up.

# Blood Loss or Overall Health?

It goes without saying that if blood loss results in women feeling exhausted in the weeks after birth, this is detrimental to both mother and child. However, haematologist, Gill Gyte (1992) suggested that it would be more useful to consider haematological and physical implications of third stage management than blood loss. She also suggested that healthy women appear to cope well with blood losses of up to 1000 mls, and that we know very little about the consequences of either very small or heavy blood loss during third stage.

There has been a growing tendency towards redefining normal blood loss. 1000 mls is not thought to be necessarily excessive in a well-nourished healthy population, providing the woman appears well (World Health Organization 1996). Midwife, Tricia Anderson (1999) recently reiterated the question of what effects there may be (if any) of reducing blood loss after birth to below the physiological norm.

Around the same time as the Bristol trial, a midwife carried out a small, retrospective research project involving 100 women at a hospital in England. She found that haemoglobin levels after three days were similar amongst the women in the trial and concluded that a physiological third stage is appropriate for some women (Watson 1990).

**41**

At the time of the research this hospital already had a physiological third stage rate of 17%. This research was important for two reasons:

* it used haemoglobin levels rather than blood loss as a term of reference. Women's health is, in fact, more important than the actual blood loss, and research shows that estimates of blood loss are frequently inaccurate, and the greater the blood loss the less accurate estimates become. The tendency is often towards underestimation when blood loss is high, and overestimation when blood loss is low. (Razvi et al 1996)

* the hospital practised physiological third stage so that midwives there were already competent and confident with this approach

# Dublin and Brighton Trials

These two trials included women who were considered to be well, and were at low risk of postpartum haemorrhage at the beginning of labour.

The Dublin trial carried out by midwife, Cecily Begley in Ireland (1990), showed much lower incidences of postpartum haemorrhage in the physiological arm of the trial than in the Bristol study. There were more retained placentas (and therefore manual removals of placentas) in the group of women who had actively managed third stages of labour. There were side effects of Ergometrine including raised blood pressure, nausea and vomiting in some women, but intravenous Ergometrine was the oxytocic used.

In the small Brighton trial (Thiliganathan et al 1993) the main findings were that there was no difference in blood loss between the two groups of women having physiological or active management of the third stage (though this was estimated only) - but more significantly, three days after birth, haemoglobin levels were similar in the two groups. The third stage of labour in this trial was found to be longer in the group of women in the physiological arm of the trial.

# Hinchingbrooke Trial

In the early 1990s, many of those involved in discussions about third stage management saw the need for further research. Gill Gyte discussed how this could be taken forward in an excellent article, entitled, 'Evaluation of the meta-analysis on the effects on both mother and baby, of the various components of active management of the third stage of labour' (Gyte 1994). At this time, further research was already being designed.

Based on their own practice and the desire for knowledge amongst women, researchers planned and carried out the Hinchingbrooke trial (Rogers & Wood 1999). This study aimed to answer questions the Bristol trial and other research had been unable to do. It was unusual in that it took place in a hospital setting where physiological third stage for healthy women having normal labours was not uncommon.

The trial concluded that the rate of PPH was two and half times greater in the group of women assigned to the physiological arm of the trial compared with the group of women who received active management (16.5% in the physiological group compared with 6.8% in the active management group, i.e., 10 women need to have active management to prevent one PPH). There was no difference in the number of retained placentas.

The trial also confirmed the side-effects of Syntometrine in the group of women given Syntometrine to expel the placenta. The babies of the women who had physiological third stages were slightly heavier - probably because of the extra blood they received whilst the cord was still pulsating after birth (Rogers & Wood 1999, Rogers et al 1998).

Curiously, from 1986-1988, at this same hospital, the PPH rate was 7% in the group of women who had physiological third stages, compared to a 7.6% overall rate (Levy 1990).

# Systematic Reviews

Most recently, the findings of the four randomised trials (Brighton, Bristol, Dublin and Hinchingbrooke) have been combined in a systematic review on the Cochrane Library. This database provides systematic reviews of all randomised controlled trials deemed to be of good quality in maternity care. A systematic review pools together the data from similar research trials. Researchers concluded that:

"...the data suggests that in the setting of a maternity hospital, active management is consistently associated with:

- a reduced risk of maternal blood loss, PPH and severe PPH, prolonged third stage of labour and maternal anaemia.

- an increased risk of maternal nausea, vomiting and raised blood pressure (almost certainly because all four trials utilised Ergometrine as a component of the oxytocic drug used), and

**45**

- no apparent advantages or disadvantages to the baby. (Prendiville 1998; see also Anderson 1999 for further comment). Though the long-term effects on the baby have not been evaluated."

It is perhaps debatable whether it is useful and informative to combine trials as different as some of these trials were. Interestingly, it is still unclear which component of active management reduces blood loss (Rogers & Wood 1999).

# Other Research and Alternative Views

A worrying factor which came to light in a relatively recent piece of research is the impact of the individual practitioner on the occurrence of postpartum haemorrhage. It was discovered that, in a particular hospital, the postpartum haemorrhage rates varied from 1-16% for midwives, and 1-31% for registrars. Doctors and midwives considered to be 'heavy-handed', had much higher rates (Logue, 1990). No subsequent research has been carried out, despite the fact that this seems to be an important finding.

As mentioned previously, Odent provides a very different analysis of the third stage of labour. A study in New Zealand (Prichard et al 1995) may lend support to Odent's argument. 213 women who had home births were included in the study. The emphasis was on the lack of disturbance to the physiological processes of birth, and showed few women had postpartum haemorrhages (3.3%). None of the women required a manual removal of the placenta. Interestingly, the lengths of the first, second and third stages of labour bore no relation to blood loss.

There was a tendency for women with higher haemoglobin counts in late pregnancy to lose more blood after birth, and 15% of the women who had had previous postpartum haemorrages had a subsequent one. Crucially, no woman had a reported blood loss of more than 900ml - however the researchers acknowledged that estimated blood loss can be inaccurate and that the methods used in this research may have introduced bias. They conclude that it raised important issues for exploration rather than providing definitive answers.

There are also concerns about the baby, which have not been accepted by many professionals but which should be topics for further research. Dunn suggests that actively managing the third stage of labour affects the adaptation of the newborn to extrauterine life, particularly in a preterm baby born by caesarean section (Dunn 1991). He has developed an approach designed to avoid the iatrogenic (medically induced) consequences of active management of the third stage. This includes leaving the cord pulsating after birth (Dunn 1991, Dunn 1989).

# Further Questions To Be Asked

There are still questions to be asked, and it is now acknowledged that defining a postpartum haemorrhage as a blood loss of over 500ml in healthy, well-nourished women may be inappropriate. It has been suggested that a cut off point of 500mls is not based on robust scientific evidence, but is a pragmatic definition based on the 'currency of the day' (Rogers 1998, personal communication). This 'day' was some time ago, when many women were less healthy and gave birth to many babies.

Defining retained placenta in terms of time limits may also be misleading (Prichard et al 1995). Redefining postpartum haemorrhage as a blood loss of over 1000mls for example, and extending or removing time limits from the third stage would considerably alter the interpretation of research results to date, and alter research design in the future. New Zealand midwife, Kirsty Prichard, along with others, suggests that 'an assessment of the woman's physiological response to the blood loss' be considered (Prichard 1995). Researchers also suggest that trials should be carried out in other settings, especially in the home, as there appear to be different practices and outcomes in this setting.

An ongoing randomised controlled trial in the Netherlands on the management of the third stage of labour, the LENTE trial, will provide us with further valuable information as it includes women having home births. The results should be available in due course (Herschderfer 1999, personal communication). Active management of the third stage of labour is not necessarily routinely recommended in the Netherlands and according to de Groot et al (1996) only 10% of midwives and 55% of obstetricians routinely used oxytocics for third stage management. Also, in that country, postpartum haemorrhage is defined as a blood loss of 1000 mls or more.

One of the interesting criticisms of the randomised controlled trials to date, is that in all groups in the trials, the third stage is in fact 'managed'. (Odent 1998b). Odent suggests that expectant third stage management is defined in negative terms in relation to active management, i.e. it is an avoidance of active management. It has not been defined in positive terms, i.e. factors that may promote the safety and efficiency of a natural third stage. He believes that the research is therefore biased towards managed third stage from the outset and that disturbance to the physiological processes have a major influence on the third stage. He claims that in the randomised trials to date, these are 'highly disturbed both in the study groups and the control groups' (Odent 1998b).

In addition, one of the main problems identified by Gill Gyte (1994) has still not been addressed in any of the research to date - that is, when a woman having a physiological third stage requires treatment, she often

**49**

receives a "mix and match" (a mixture of both physiological and active management) approach, rather than moving to active management (see Gyte 1998 and National Childbirth Trust 1993).

It could thus still be argued that the research to date shows that in a busy maternity unit, where a woman is unlikely to be completely undisturbed during childbirth, where time limits are likely to be imposed, and where midwives are more familiar with active management, routinely recommending, active management of the third stage of labour reduces blood loss after birth and may thus be preferable to many women. This raises many questions and ethical issues about the management of birth in Britain and elsewhere, and how women can be supported to experience physiological births in large obstetric units.

One of the problems with basing practice purely on scientific research, especially randomised controlled trials, is that it can disregard crucial experiential and observational knowledge. Well-designed, and expertly carried out research trials can give us good information about treatments and practices involving large groups of people, but tell us little about individuals - the differences between people and the subtle affects of treatments and procedures. Experiential and observational knowledge often provides the basis for more systematic research, but also tells us about individuals and practices which may be less easily measured by quantitative, scientific research.

For example, some of the most experienced midwives in Britain and other westernised countries do not recommend the routine use of Syntometrine for the third stage of labour. They do, however, emphasise the need to develop an ongoing relationship with women, so that amongst other issues, they can consider the likelihood of the woman bleeding after birth and can take steps in pregnancy to reduce any risks - possibly through effective dietary or lifestyle changes. There is a need for continuity of carer and the development of mutual understanding so that the woman and midwife can work together during labour and birth to optimise the likelihood of all going well. In the unlikely event of bleeding occurring unexpectedly, this trust enables them to work together efficiently and deal with the emergency as safely and quickly as possible (see for example, a collection of articles in a recent *Midwifery Today* journal on 'Haemorrhage' 1998 and Welsh 1997).

Midwives practising this way rely on scientific evidence to guide their practice. They also use their own experiential knowledge, and that of others, which has usually been gained over many years. Whilst they expect birth to unfold safely, they are alert at all times, to the possibility of unexpected changes, which may require rapid and efficient responses. They also heed their intuition, and because the relationship with the woman is central to their practice, they are attuned to the women in their care.

One midwife described an unusual incident of a woman having a velamentous insertion of the cord (where the vessels of the cord separate and go through the membranes before reaching the placenta).

The midwife knew the woman, knew that the pattern of her labour was unusual and encouraged her to follow her instincts despite the unusually slow, stop-start progress of her labour. She was reminded of Australian GP, John Stevenson's observation that this can be a sign of the body taking care of a problem with the cord - such as a knot.

The midwife refrained from intervening with the normal course of labour and the baby was born healthy and well. Only after the arrival of the placenta was the midwife able to understand the problem. It is possible that any of the standard medical interventions for a 'prolonged' labour could have seriously compromised the baby and may even have been fatal (Wolford 1997).

It seems we still have some way to go in balancing different forms of knowledge, and have much to learn from midwives and doctors who have incorporated an openness to different ways of knowing in their own practices and who listen to women, observe carefully, and treat each woman as an individual.

# A Difficult Decision?

Given the inconclusive results and varied interpretation of scientific research, and considered alternative knowledge, how can the individual woman make an informed decision about whether to accept or decline the active or physiological approach to the third stage of labour? Three important considerations seem to be:

- the difficulty in defining a physiological third stage of labour

- the poor ability to identify women at risk of developing problems during this phase of birth with any accuracy

- how best to make information available to help women to them make their own decision

There are suggested risk factors associated with third stage problems. Whilst this list is not definitive, these include having:

- known blood clotting disorders - women who bruise or bleed easily or who have particularly heavy periods should be tested antenatally and active management may be appropriate (Gyte, personal communication)

**53**

- antepartum haemorrhage

- third stage problems in a previous labour

- anaemia

- a multiple birth

- a prolonged labour

- a precipitate labour

- oxytocic drugs during labour - if the woman's labour has been induced or accelerated with an oxytocic drip, the drip should be left in place until after the placenta is born

None of the above would automatically cause problems and it is essential that when a woman intends to avoid the use of oxytocic drugs she is able to discuss this fully with a midwife who is knowledgeable and confident about this preference.

Research shows that women often know little about the third stage of labour (Green et al 1998). As the issues are complex, each woman should be able to talk about the third stage with a midwife and receive full and balanced information during her pregnancy. Women should not be expected to consider the pros and cons of physiological versus active management for the first time during labour or after the baby's birth.

It should be acknowledged that women will use information and interpret research in different ways, which fit in with their personal values and attitudes. They should be respected and supported. This issues is and will continue to be problematic if policies in place recommend active management, but midwives are expected to provide choice.

At Hinchingbrooke Hospital, where the latest third stage trial was carried out, the researchers commented that 'when physiological management is offered to women as a reasonable option, many will choose it' - of those women who could have taken part in the study, 52% chose physiological management, and 39% chose active management during the trial (Rogers and Wood 1999).

# How A Woman Feels During the Third Stage

Whilst defining labour in terms of different stages may be helpful, there is a danger that we lose sight of the process of birth and apply principles out of context, failing to recognise the inter-relatedness of the whole process.

How birth unfolds has direct and indirect implications for the relationship between mother and baby, and how the mother feels about herself. This holds true of the third stage, as at any other time during

**55**

birth. It can be a particularly delicate and awesome time, as the mother sees her baby for the first time and, if all is well, is able slowly to come to terms with this and get to know her baby. Whether the woman and her attendants have decided to manage the third stage actively or passively, the atmosphere remains crucial.

A calm, unhurried environment will encourage the mother to get to know her baby in her own time and in her own way. She may want to pick the baby up and put it to her breast, or let the baby begin to take in his/her surroundings, and gaze into her eyes. Whilst the term 'bonding' may have become a cliché, the concept is vital in promoting a healthy start to parenting. It is an ongoing process and is highly significant around the time of birth. Any approach should therefore seek to minimise interference at this time.

For women, the birthing of the placenta may be quick and easy, taking minutes, or it may take a good deal longer. Very occasionally the woman may feel discomfort or pain which can be intense and distressing. Some women may still feel over-awed by the birth or feel exhausted, cold, shivery, detached or confused, whilst others are keen to 'get it over with', feeling tired and anxious to put the birth behind them so as to be able to focus on their newborn baby. For some women it is important to allow the third stage to unfold in its own time and to have a sense of completion, before moving their focus of attention to the baby.

There is no 'right' way to give birth and, at any stage of labour, any routine intervention is not without its risks. Good communication between the mother and her attendant is an important component for the mother and the baby's well-being and, whilst controversy surrounds management of the third stage of labour, it is particularly important that a mutual understanding exists (see Green et al, 1998). In asking the question "what is the 'best'" care, policy-makers and care givers should accept that part of the answer lies in providing individualised care for individual women based on their preferences and individual circumstances

# Further Reading

Cronk M, Flint C (1989) Community Midwifery - A Practical Guide, Heinemann Medical Books

Enkin M, Kierse MJNC, Nielson J, Renfrew M (1995) A Guide to Effective Care in Pregnancy and Childbirth, Second Edition, Oxford University Press

Inch S (1989) Birthrights, Greenprint

Priya JV (1992) Modern Care in Pregnancy and Childbirth, Element

National Childbirth Trust (1993) The Third Stage of Labour. Available from NCT Maternity Sales Ltd., Burnfield Ave, Glasgow, G46 7TI.

Thomas P (1996) Every Woman's Birth Rights, Thorsons

Thomas P (1997) Every Birth Is Different, Headline

# More Information

**AIMS**
Beverley Lawrence Beech
21 Iver Lane
Iver, Bucks SLO 9LH
Tel: 01753 652781

For a copy of **AIMS'** free
Publications List send s.a.e to:

Janette McCabe
1 Cortleferry Grove
Eskbank
Midlothian EH22 3HX

**MIDIRS**
(Midwife Information and
Research Service)
9 Elmdale Road
Clifton, Bristol B58 1SL
Tel: 0117-925-1791

**NCT**
(National Childbirth Trust)
Alexander House
Oldham Terrace
London W3 6NH
Tel: 0181 992 8637

# References

Anderson T (1998) *Prophylactic syntometrine vs oxytocin in the third stage of labour,* Practising Midwife, Vol 1 No 10. p40-41

Anderson T (1999) *Active versus expectant management of the third stage of labour,* Practising Midwife, Vol 2 No 2 p 10-11

Begley CM (1990) *A comparison of 'active' and 'physiological' management of the third stage of labour,* Midwifery, Vol 6 No 1, p3-17

Begley CM (1990) *The effect of ergometrine on breastfeeding,* Midwifery, Vol 6 No 2 PAGE

Botha MC (1968) *The management of the umbilical cord in labour,* South African Journal of Obstetrics and Gynaecology Vol 16 No 2, p30-33

Chalmers I (1990) *Care during the third stage of labour,* Commentary on a Commentary, AIMS Quarterly Journal Vol 2 No 3 p8-11

Cronk M, Flint C (1989) *Community Midwifery: A Practical Guide,* Heinemann Medical Books, Chapter 4 p50-71

de Groot ANJA, van Roosmalen J, van Dongen PWJ (1996) *Survey of the management of third stage of labour in the Netherlands,* European Journal of Obstetrics and Gynaecology and Reproductive Biology, vol 66, p 39-40

Department of Health (1998) *Why mothers die: report on confidential enquiries into maternal deaths in the United Kingdom, 1994-6,* London: HMSO

Dewhurst J (1990) *The prevention of postpartum haemorrhage: A Review,* Journal of Obstetrics and Gynaecology, Vol 10 Suppl 2

van Dongen PWJ, de Groot ANJA (1995) *History of ergot alkaloids from ergotism to ergometrine,* European Journal of Obstetrics and Gynaecology and Reproductive Biology, Vol 60 No2, p 109-116

Dunn PM (1991) *The third stage of labour and fetal adaptation at birth,* Wyeth Guest Lecture, 1st International Congress of Perinatal Medicine, Tokyo, November 7

Dunn PM (1989) *Perinatal factors influencing adaptation to extrauterine life.* In: *Advances in Gynaecology and Obstetrics,* Vol 5, Pregnancy and Labour. Proc. 12th World Congr. Obstet. Gynec., Rio de Janeiro, Oct. (1988) Ed by Belfort P, Pinotti JA and Eskes TKAB. Parthenon Publ, Carnforth Lancs 15, p119-123

Dunn PM (1985) *Management of childbirth in normal women. The third stage and fetal adaption.* In: *Perinatal medicine.* Proceedings of the IX European Congress Perinatal Medicine, Dublin, September 1984. MTP Press, Chapter 7, 47-54

Dunn PM, Frazer ID, Raper AB (1966) *Influence of early cord ligation on the transplacental passage of the foetal cells,* Journal of Obstetrics and Gynaecology of the British Commonwealth, 73, p757-760

Enkin M, Kierse MJNC, Chalmers I (1991) *A Guide to Effective Care in Pregnancy and Childbirth,* Oxford University Press, Chapter 36

Enkin M, Kierse MJNC, Nielson J, Renfrew M (1995) *A Guide to Effective Care in Pregnancy and Childbirth, Second Edition,* Oxford University Press

Fadiman, A (1997) *The spirit catches you and you fall down - a Hmong child, her American doctors and the collision of two cultures,* New York: Farrar, Straus and Giroux

Featherstone IE (1999) *Physiological third stage of labour,* British Journal of Midwifery, Vol 7: 4, p216-221

Green JM, Coupland VA, Kitzinger JV (1998) *Great expectations: a prospective study of women's expectations and experiences of childbirth,* Books for Midwives Press, Vol 2 Chapter 6 p 322-347

Gulmezoglu AM (1998) *Prostaglandins for the management for the third stage of labour* (Cochrane Review) In: *The Cochrane Library,* Issue 4 Oxford. Update Software

Gyte G (1998) *Informed choice and the third stage of labour,* Research Matters No 7. Available from NCT

Gyte G (1994) *Evaluation of the meta-analysis on the effects on both mother and baby, of the various components of 'active management' of the third stage of labour,* Midwifery, Vol. 10, p183-199

Gyte G (1992) *The significance of blood loss at delivery*, MIDIRS Midwifery Digest, Vol. 2, No. 1, p88-92

Gyte G (1990) The continuing debate on the third stage of labour, AIMS Quarterly Journal, Vol. 3, No. 1, p4-6

Gyte G (1990) *The Bristol third stage trial*, Teachers' Broadsheet, New Generation, Vol. 9, No. 1, p29

Harding JE, Elbourne DA, Prendiville PJ (1989) *Views of mothers and midwives participating in the Bristol randomised controlled trial of active management of the third stage of labour*, Birth Vol. 16, No. 1, p1-6

Hemminki E, Marilainen J (1996) *Long term effects of caesarean sections: ectopic pregnancies and placental problems*, Am J Ob Gyn, 174: 1569-73

Herschderfer K (1999) Personal Communication

Hunt, S and Symonds A (1995) *The Social Meaning of Midwifery*, London: Macmillan

Inch S (1990) *Bristol third stage trial commentary*, AIMS Quarterly Journal, Vol 1, No. 4, p8-10

Inch S *Birthrights* (1989) Greenprint Chapter 7, p145-191

Inch S (1985) *Management of the third stage of labour - another cascade of intervention?* Midwifery 1(2): 114-112

Inch S (1983) *Third stage management*, Association of Radical Midwives Newsletter, No. 19, p7-8

Kierse MJNC (1998) *What does prevent postpartum haemorrhage?*, Lancet 351, March 7, p690-692

Kloosterman G (1975) In: *Immaculate Deception* by Arms S, Houghton Mifflin

Lapido OA (1971) *Management of third stage of labour with particular reference to reduction of feto-maternal transfusion*, British Medical Journal, 18 March , pp 721-723

Levy V (1990) *The midwife's management of the third stage of labour*, In Alexander J, Levy V, and Roch S (eds) Midwifery Practice: *Intrapartum Care - A Research Based Approach*, Macmillan

Levy V, Moore J (1985) *The midwife's management of the third stage of labour*, Nursing Times, Vol. 81, No. 5, p 47-50

Lewis V et al (1998) *Why mothers die: report on a confidential enquiry into maternal deaths in the United Kingdom* 1994-1996, London HMSO

Logue M (1990) *Management of the third stage of labour: a midwife's view*, Journal of Obstetrics and Gynaecology, Vol. 10, Suppl. 2, p 10-12

McDonald S, Prendiville WJ, Elbourne DA (1999) *Prophylactic syntometrine versus oxytocin for delivery of the placenta* (Cochrane Review; last updated: 17 Oct 1996. In: The Cochrane Library Issue 2, Oxford: Update Software

McDonald SJ, Prendiville W, Blair E (1993) *Randomised controlled trial of oxytocin alone versus oxytocin and ergometrine in active management of the third stage of labour*, British Medical Journal 307, p1167-1171

Midwifery Today (1998) *Haemorrhage* Special Edition, No 48

National Childbirth Trust (1993) *The third stage of labour* (available from the NCT)

Odent M (1998a) *Physiological birth is normal birth*, Midwifery Today Conference 'Keeping Birth Normal', London. Sept 10-14

Odent M (1998b) *Don't manage the third stage of labour!* Practising Midwife; 1: 9, p31-33

Peyser MR, Kupfermine MJ (1990) *Management of severe postpartum haemorrhage by intrauterine irrigation with prostaglandin E2*, American Journal of Obstetrics and Gynaecology, Vol 1, No. 3

Porter M, MacIntyre S (1984) *What is must be best: a research note on conservative or deferential responses to antenatal care provision*, Soc. Sci. Med Vol 9: 11. p 1197-1200

Prendiville WJ, Elbourne DA, McDonald S (1999) *Active versus expectant management of the third stage of labour*, (Cochrane Review; last updated 8 July 1998). In: *The Cochrane Library*, Issue 2. Oxford: Update Software

Prendiville W, Elbourne D (1989) *Care during the third stage of labour*, In Chalmers I, Enkin M, Kierse MJNC (eds) *Effective Care in Pregnancy and Childbirth*, Oxford University Press. Vol 2 p 1145-1169

Prendiville WJ, Harding, JE, Elbourne DA (1988) *The Bristol third stage trial: active versus physiological management of third stage labour*, British Medical Journal, Vol. 297, p1295-1300

Prichard K, O'Boyle A, Hogden J (1995) *Third stage of labour: outcomes of physiological third stage of labour care in the homebirth setting (November 1991)*, New Zealand College of Midwives Journal, April, 8-10

Priya JV (1992) *Modern Care in Pregnancy and Childbirth*, Element

Razvi K, Chua S, Arulkumaran S, Ratman SS (1996). *A comparison between visual estimation of laboratory determination of blood loss during the third stage of labour*, Australian and New Zealand Journal of Obstetrics and Gynaecology, Vol 36 No 2, p152-154

Rogers J (1998) Letter to the author

Rogers J, Wood J (1999) *The Hinchingbrooke third stage trial: what are the implications for practice*, Practising Midwife Vol 2 No 2, p35-37

Rogers J, Wood J, McCandlish R, Ayers S, Truesdale A, Elbourne D (1998) *Active versus expectant management of third stage of labour: the Hinchingbrooke randomised controlled trial*, Lancet Vol 351 March 7, p693-699

Santalahti P et al (1998) *On what grounds to women participate in prenatal screening?* Prenatal Diagnosis, Vol 18, No 2, p153-165

Sleep J (1993) *Physiology and management of the third stage of labour*, In Bennet VR Brown IK (eds) *Myles Textbook for Midwives* (12th edition), Churchill Livingstone, Chapter 15, p216-229

Stevenson J (1989) *The Bristol third stage trial* Association of Radical Midwives Magazine, No. 4, p11-12

Stockdale H (1997) *Overview of the management of the third stage of labour,* Open Line Vol 5 No 3, p 9-10, 21-22

Sweet BR (1997) *Midwifery care in the third stage of labour,* In Sweet BR (ed) *Mayes' Midwifery: A Textbook for Midwives* (12th Ed) Balliere Tindall. Chapter 31, p403-417

Thilaganathan B, Cutner A, Latimer J, Beard R (1993) *Management of the third stage of labour in women at low risk of postpartum haemorrhage,* European Journal of Obstetrics and Gynaecology and Reproductive Biology; Vol 48 No 1, p19-22

Ward A (1983) *Syntometrine,* Association of Radical Midwives Newsletter, No. 18, p21-25

Watson B (1990) *A study of haemoglobin levels in women before and after childbirth,* Midwives Chronicle, vol 103, no 1228, p156-158

Welsh G (1997) *Wisdom of the midwives: postpartum bleeding,* Midwifery Today No 42, p 13

Wesson N (1990) *Homebirth,* London, Macdonald Optima

Wood J, Rogers J (1997). *The third stage of labour.* In: Alexander J, Levy V, Roth C (eds). *Midwifery Practice: Core Topics 2,* Macmillan Press Ltd, p 113-126.

Wolford MC (1997) *First do no harm,* Midwifery Today, p15-17

World Health Organization (1996) *Care in normal birth: a practical guide,* Report of a Technical Working Group, WHO/FRH/MSM/96.24, Geneva

Yoa AC, Lind J (1974) *Placental transfusion,* American Journal of Diseases in Children vol 127, p128-141

Zaki M et al (1998) *Risk factors and morbidity in patients with placenta previa accreta compared to placenta previa non-accreta,* Acta Obstetrica Gynecologica Scandinavia, vol 77, p391-94